HEALTHFUL ESSENCE COOKBOOK
Caribbean-Style Vegan Vegetarian Meals

Healthful Essence Cookbook

Caribbean-Style Vegan Vegetarian Meals

Princess Rowena Daly-Dixon

ATLANTA 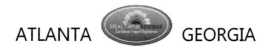 GEORGIA

Healthful Essence Cookbook
Caribbean-Style Vegan Vegetarian Meals
By, Princess Rowena Daly-Dixon

Copyright © 2011 by Princess Rowena Daly-Dixon
Library of Congress Control Number: 2011930471
ISBN-10: 061551314X
ISBN-13: 978-0-615-51314-0

Published by
Healthful Essence
875 York Avenue, SW
Atlanta, GA 30310
www.healthfullessence.com
princessdixon20@msn.com
(404) 806-0830

Book Editing:
Betty Thompson, Dr. Serwaa Ajanaku (aka Silvia Walker), and Abena Muhammad
Page Layout and Cover Design:
Abena Muhammad, DetailsCount@yahoo.com
Cover and Inside Photography:
Abena Muhammad, DetailsCount@yahoo.com
Food Styling:
Princess Daly-Dixon and Charles Dixon

10 9 8 7 6 5 4 3 2 1
First Printing

PRINTED IN THE U.S.A.

This book is dedicated

to my son, **Charles**, *who has been*

working with me from the age of six years

and my daughter, **Donna**, *who gave me*

the strength and help to carry on.

FOREWORD

Most of us enjoy a hearty breakfast. For many of us, this breakfast has been passed down from generation to generation—often since the days of slavery. If the breakfast of our parents included an abundance of fat, sugar, butter and salt, more than likely we will prepare our morning meal in the same manner. Unfortunately, the diet we enjoyed as youths and continue to enjoy with our own families, has contributed to the many illnesses such as diabetes, high blood pressure, heart disease, low energy, and premature aging that negatively affect African American health.

Many of us would like to change our diet but do not know where to begin. The first step towards a healthier diet, is as easy as drinking a glass of our "Morning Sunshine Cocktail." Just squeeze a teaspoon of fresh lemon in a glass of spring or filtered water upon rising to help rid the body of impurities. Pure water is the first step towards good health and should be consumed first thing every morning.

We are living in a time of severe health challenges and deterioration and the foods we consume greatly contribute to our state of health. The meat and dairy free recipes found in our Healthful Essence Cookbook are not only nutritious, but easy to prepare, and very satisfying to the taste. We hope you enjoy these tasty recipes and wish you good health through nutritious foods.

CONTENTS

INTRODUCTION

I was born in Kitty Village in the beautiful land of Guyana, South America. I have always enjoyed tasty foods and their presentation. At the age of nine my duty was to prepare food for our family. This essential duty lasted until I turned nineteen and decided to travel to London, England.

I spent nine years in London. While there, I married a Jamaican and we subsequently left London to live in Jamaica. In 1982, I traveled to the United States, and continued to seek knowledge on the preparation, combination and presentation of vegetarian cuisine. While in New York, I was introduced to the study of Microcosmic Science (a study of the inhabitant of the community of the body) under the leader and founder, Dr. Ignatius Foster. The knowledge gained from this study helped me to develop culinary skills that encouraged the formation and maintenance of a healthy lifestyle through the preparation of healthy foods.

My classmates and I started a small business preparing and selling foods at carnivals, fetes and annual festivals. I was the head cook. Patrons enjoyed our food tremendously. We received a great number of positive responses from non-vegetarians and vegetarian customers alike. This experience helped me to realize that I could make a living from the food business. I bought a new Chevy Van and a food cart and used them to start my own food business near the World Trade Center in Manhattan, New York. I operated this business from 1989 to 1998. It was a pleasure to hear how well customers enjoyed my food.

I then moved to Atlanta and opened a vegetarian restaurant called Healthful Essence, which is currently in operation today. It was at that time that I first developed the Healthful Essence Vegetarian Cookbook which also includes recipes from Sister Sylvia Rowe. Written communication is a very effective way to reach people and encourage them to change or improve their diet.

I have been a vegetarian for twenty-three years now and I have experienced remarkable improvement in my level of energy. My thinking is much sharper and I have consistency keeping my weight balanced. It is clear to me that eating healthy, well-prepared, fresh foods can make a big difference in the way a person thinks, feels and acts. I experienced no problems during menopause and I attribute this successful passage to my Healthful Essence Vegetarian Diet—which is based mainly on recipes presented in this cookbook. These recipes, including my desserts and refreshing drinks, are natural, simple, nutritious, and easy to prepare, yet unbelievably satisfying and pleasing to the palate.

We are living in a time of severe health deterioration (dis-ease) in America and throughout the world. Thus, there is an urgent need—now more than ever before—for the health conscious among us to maintain a vigilant eye on intelligent selection of food, healthy eating, full body cleansing and sensible weight control. I encourage you to start your holistic nutritional journey by trying the delicious main courses, entrees, desserts and drinks, in my Healthful Essence Cookbook.

To your health,
Princess Rowena Daly-Dixon

PART 1
Good Morning, Good Breakfast

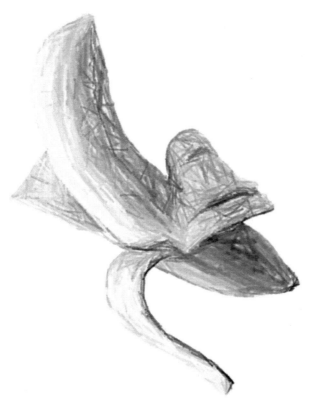

Green Banana Porridge

INGREDIENTS

1 large or 2 med	green bananas
1 stick	cinnamon
2 cups	filtered water
5 whole	cloves
2 Tbsp	brown sugar or sweetener of your choice
2 drops	almond extract
1 pinch	nutmeg
1 pinch	sea salt

DIRECTIONS

1. Wash bananas, cut off ends. Cut into small pieces peeled or unpeeled.

2. Put 1 cup of filtered water into blender. Add small pieces of banana and blend until fine.

3. Boil 2 cups of water with cinnamon stick, cloves and salt for 10 minutes.

4. Add blended banana to boiled, spiced water. Stir until mixture begins to get thick. Lower heat and let simmer for 5 minutes.

5. Add rest of ingredients. Stir again and shut off stove.

6. This can be served with soy milk, almond milk or coconut milk.

Stoneground Cornmeal Porridge

INGREDIENTS

½ cup	cornmeal
1 stick	cinnamon
5 whole	cloves
1 pinch	sea salt
1 ½ cups	spring or filtered water
3 drops	almond extract
2 Tbsp	brown sugar or sweetener
3 drops	vanilla extract
1 pinch	nutmeg

DIRECTIONS

1. Soak cornmeal in ½ cup water.
2. Boil 1 cup of water with cinnamon stick, clove and sea salt.
3. Add soaked cornmeal. Boil for 10 minutes.
4. Add remaining ingredients. Sweeten to taste.
5. Serve with almond, soy or coconut milk.

Raw Oatmeal Cereal

INGREDIENTS

½ cup	stoneground oatmeal, soaked
1 Tbsp	pumpkin seed
1 Tbsp	sunflower seed
1 ½ cups	water
1 dash	nutmeg
1 dash	cinnamon
1 Tbsp	almond nuts
1 Tbsp	wheat germ
1–2 Tbsp	brown sugar, maple syrup or honey to taste

DIRECTIONS

1. Soak nuts. Blend all ingredients together.
2. Sweeten to taste, sprinkle wheat germ on top and serve.

Potato Scallion Pancakes

INGREDIENTS

1 lb	potatoes
½ stalk	leek
2 sprigs	scallion
1 pinch	basil
1 clove	garlic
1 pinch	sea salt

DIRECTIONS

1. Shred potatoes, mince garlic and leeks. Add salt to taste.
2. Drop by spoonfuls and bake on grill.

Oatmeal Pancakes

INGREDIENTS

1 cup	oatmeal, quick cooking
¼ cup	wheat germ
¼ cup	soy, almond or milk of your choice
1 tsp	baking soda
1 pinch	salt
1 Tbsp	brown sugar
1 cup	water
1 tsp	egg replacer
1 Tbsp	margarine

DIRECTIONS

1. Combine all ingredients and stir until blended.
2. Bake on grill.

Journey Cakes (Bakes)
Fried Dumplings

INGREDIENTS

¼ cup	unbleached flour
½ cup	whole wheat flour
1 tsp	sea salt
1 Tbsp	soy margarine
1 tsp	baking powder (aluminum free)
1 Tbsp	brown sugar (optional)
	a little cold water
	oil for frying

DIRECTIONS

1. Mix flour and baking powder together and pass through sieve.

2. Chop in margarine, salt and sugar. Mix to a firm dough with sufficient water to make it easy to roll out.

3. Roll ½ inch thick. Cut in rounds with a small glass or cup and fry in deep oil.

Scrambled Tofu

INGREDIENTS

8 oz	tofu
1 tsp	turmeric
1 Tbsp	nutritional yeast
2 stalks	scallion
4 stalks	cilantro, finely diced
¼ cup	red pepper, diced
¼ cup	green pepper, diced
2 Tbsp	corn oil
1 pinch	thyme, fresh or dried
2 cloves	garlic, diced
2 small	plum tomatoes, diced
1 pinch	cayenne
	salt to taste

DIRECTIONS

1. Crush tofu and squeeze out most of the water.
2. Sauté all other ingredients in corn oil.
3. Add tofu and cook for 10 minutes and serve.

PART 2
Dinner Delights

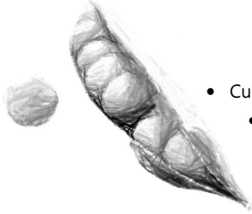

- Lentil and Barley Stew
- Vegetable Mafe'
- Stuffed Eggplant with Tofu
- Vegetarian Red Bean Chili with Caribbean Flavor
- Potato and Onion Casserole
- Millet Loaf
- Greens with Garlic
- Lentil Salad with Scallions
- Curried Chickpea (Garbanzo Beans)
- Lima Bean Stew with Pumpkin
- Millet Delight
- UnMeat Loaf
- Chickpea Loaf
- Cauliflower and Broccoli Au Gratin
- Vegetable Quiche' with Tofu
- Vegetarian Delight
- Tofu Cutlets
- Stewed Vegetable Chunks
- Curried Potatoes and Carrots
- Baked Chickette
- TVP Vegetable Medley

Cous Cous Medley •

BBQ Tofu •

Three Bean Burger •

Vegan Macaroni Uncheese •

Chickpea Patties •

Vegetable Pie •

Tofu Stir Fry •

Vegetable Lo Mein •

Coconut Curry Vegetables •

Brown Rice and Peas •

Princess's Yellow Rice •

Spicy Squash Stew •

Lentil & Barley Stew

INGREDIENTS

2 Tbsp	peanut oil
1/3 cup	onion, chopped
2 cloves	garlic, chopped
½ cup	celery, chopped
2 ½ cups	fresh tomatoes, chopped
2 cups	water
½ cup	dried lentils, picked and washed
1/3 cup	organic whole barley
¼ tsp	cayenne pepper
1/8 tsp	rosemary
½ tsp	sage
1/3 cup	diced carrots
½ tsp	sea salt

DIRECTIONS

1. Boil lentils and barley until tender.
2. Sauté onion, celery garlic, carrots, tomatoes, rosemary, sage, and sea salt.
3. Add to barley and lentil mixture.
4. Simmer for 10 minutes.
5. Turn off stove and add cayenne pepper.

Vegetable Mafe'

INGREDIENTS

1 small	onion, finely chopped
2 Tbsp	palm oil
2 cups	pumpkin, winter squash or sweet potatoes, peeled and chopped in 1-inch bits
4 med	turnips
4 med	potatoes (quartered)
2 large	carrots (cut in 1 inch bits)
½ small	cabbage, coarsely chopped (optional)
2 large	tomatoes (quartered)
1 bunch	fresh leafy greens
1 dozen	okras
2	chili peppers (or 1 tsp cayenne pepper)
2 cups	organic tomato sauce
¾ cup	organic peanut butter
2 cups	spring water

DIRECTIONS

1. Sauté onions in moderately hot oil in a large, heavy skillet or stew pot.

2. Add vegetables one at a time, sautéing each for 1 minute before adding another.

3. Stir in tomato sauce along with 2 cups of spring water.

4. Reduce heat and simmer until all vegetables are tender.

5. Spoon out about half a cup of hot broth and mix it with peanut butter to make a smooth paste. Add to pot and then add okra.

6. Simmer for another 10-15 minutes. Serve over rice.

Stuffed Eggplant
with Tofu

INGREDIENTS

2 large	eggplants (cooked whole)
1 cup	boiled brown rice
2 sprigs	fresh parsley, chopped
2 cloves	garlic, chopped
2 blades	scallions, chopped
1 sprig	fresh cilantro/coriander, chopped
1 Tbsp	cold-pressed olive oil
1 Tbsp	shoshu or Tamari sauce
1 med	red bell pepper, chopped
1 med	green bell pepper, chopped
8 oz	firm tofu (crumbled)

DIRECTIONS

1. Cook eggplant. Cut off tops of cooked eggplant. Cut down one side and carefully scoop out the meat leaving about half an inch around the walls. Drain if necessary.

2. Sauté all spices, rice, tofu, nutritional yeast and eggplant meat.

3. Stuff eggplant then slice stuffed eggplant into 1-inch slices and arrange in a shallow greased baking dish.

4. Make tomato sauce with fresh tomatoes, onion, garlic, nutritional yeast and a pinch of salt to taste.

5. Cover eggplant with tomato sauce and sprinkle with nutritional yeast, fresh minced parsley and basil.

6. Bake for 30 minutes at 350F.

Vegetarian Red Bean Chili with Caribbean Flavor

INGREDIENTS

2 cups	red beans
4 cups	water, or enough water to cook beans
¼ cup	textured vegetable protein (TVP) (optional)
1 whole	onion, chopped
1 pinch	cumin
1 pinch	turmeric
2 blades	scallion
1 sprig	fresh thyme or 1 tsp dried thyme
3 Tbsp	bread crumbs
1 pinch	brown sugar
1 pinch	sea salt
1 pinch	garlic powder
	salt to taste
	chili powder or scotch bonnet pepper to taste

DIRECTIONS

1. Boil peas until tender leaving only one cup of water after peas are tender.
2. Combine TVP, onion, scallion, thyme, cumin, turmeric, salt and pepper in a pan with a little oil.
3. Sauté until slightly brown. Add to peas and let simmer for 10 minutes.
4. Add bread crumbs and more water if needed. Add cayenne pepper.
5. Simmer for 10 more minutes and shut off stove. Serve with brown rice.

Potato and Onion Casserole

INGREDIENTS

4 large	potatoes, peeled and sliced as thin as possible
2 Tbsp	dry bread crumbs
1 ½ cups	onion, thinly sliced
2 tsp	salt (or to taste)
2 Tbsp	soy margarine or olive oil
1 Tbsp	paprika
¼ cup	soy milk
½ tsp	freshly ground pepper or scotch bonnet pepper
2 Tbsp	veggie cheese or nutritional yeast

DIRECTIONS

1. In a greased 9-inch pie dish, arrange layers of sliced potatoes and onions.
2. Sprinkle each layer with salt and pepper. Dot with one half of margarine.
3. Pour soy milk over layers. Sprinkle with bread crumbs, grated cheese, paprika and remainder of margarine.
4. Bake at 370F for 45 minutes or until potatoes are cooked.
5. Serve in pie-shaped wedges. Serves four.

Millet Loaf

INGREDIENTS

1 cup	millet (whole uncooked)
5 cups	tomato juice
1 med	onion (blended with some of tomato juice)
4 Tbsp	ground sesame seeds
½ cup	ground almonds or cashew
1 can	olives, chopped (optional)
1 tsp	sea salt
½ tsp	savory seasoning
½ tsp	sage
½ cup	celery, diced

DIRECTIONS

1. Mix all ingredients.
2. Bake in shallow, covered casserole at 325F for 2 to 5 hours or until liquid is absorbed.

Greens with Garlic

INGREDIENTS

1 bunch	mustard greens, turnip tops, kale, collard greens or broccoli robe
3 cloves	garlic
1 Tbsp	virgin olive oil
1 pinch	sea salt or Spike seasoning
1 dash	nutmeg

DIRECTIONS

1. Wash greens. Cut into small bits. Mince garlic.

2. Heat oil and add minced garlic. Sauté for one minute then add chopped greens. Add a little water if necessary and cover.

3. Cook over low flame stirring occasionally.

4. Sprinkle with salt and nutmeg. Stir.

5. Serve hot with rice or millet.

Lentil Salad with Scallions

INGREDIENTS

2 cups	lentils
1 med	onion (cut in quarters)
3 clove	garlic
1 small	bay leaf
¼ tsp	sea salt
6 cups	water (or enough to fully cover beans)
4 Tbsp	vegetable oil
1 pinch	cayenne pepper
2 Tbsp	apple cider vinegar
4	scallions, white and green parts thinly sliced
¼ cup	minced parsley
2 plum	tomatoes

DIRECTIONS

1. Wash and drain the lentils. Place lentils, onions, garlic, bay leaf, salt and water in a saucepan.

2. Bring to a boil and then lower heat to medium. Allow to simmer for 30 minutes or until lentils are tender.

3. Drain and discard the bay leaf. Place the lentils in a bowl.

4. In a screw top jar combine oil, vinegar, salt, pepper and dry mustard. Shake the jar to mix ingredients.

5. Pour over the lentils and toss lightly. Allow to cool to room temperature.

6. Just before serving, add the thinly sliced scallions and minced parsley. Season to taste.

7. Serve garnished with avocado slices and quartered tomatoes.

Curried Chick Peas
(Garbanzo Beans)

INGREDIENTS

1 cup	chick peas (boiled, cover beans with enough water to soften)
2 blades	scallion
3 cloves	garlic
1 inch	fresh ginger piece
2 small	tomatoes
1 tsp	thyme, fresh or dried
1 tsp	sea salt
1 Tbsp	Jamaican curry powder
1 tsp	cumin
1 Tbsp	peanut oil
2 small	tomatoes

DIRECTIONS

1. Boil chickpeas until tender. Strain off water and keep to be used later.
2. Chop scallions, garlic, ginger, and tomatoes.
3. Sauté in peanut oil with curry powder. Stir and add chickpeas, water and thyme.
4. Cook for 15 minutes. Add salt to taste.
5. Serve with millet or brown rice.

Lima Bean Stew with Pumpkin

INGREDIENTS

1 cup	lima beans
1 small	onion
½ med	red pepper
½ med	green pepper
2 cloves	garlic
1 cup	pumpkin, diced
1 med	carrot, cut in wedges
1 small	ginger piece
1 pinch	rosemary
1 pinch	sage
1 pinch	thyme
2	bay leaves
3	pimento seeds (whole allspice)
2 ½ cups	water
1 tsp	sea salt (or Spike seasoning)

DIRECTIONS

1. Soak and cook lima beans with pimento seeds and bay leaves until beans are soft.

2. Discard pimento seed and bay leaves.

3. Chop red pepper, green pepper, onion, garlic and add to lima beans.

4. Add remaining ingredients. Simmer for 15 minutes. Add salt to taste.
(This recipe is also delicious if you substitute the pumpkin with black squash-kombucha squash.)

Millet Delight

INGREDIENTS

1 cup	millet
2	bay leaves
1 sprig	scallion
1 clove	garlic
1 med	carrot
1 pinch	thyme
1 ½ cup	water
1 tsp	spike seasoning or sea salt
1 blade	celery
½ cup	frozen green, sweet peas
1 med	yellow squash

DIRECTIONS

1. Boil water with bay leaves. Pick and wash millet.
2. Chop garlic, carrot, scallion, thyme, yellow squash, and celery in small bits and add to water with bay leaves.
3. Add salt and let boil for 2 minutes.
4. Add millet, cover and let cook on a low fire.
5. Stir with a fork. Add more water if needed.
6. Add green peas before the millet has absorbed all the water.

Unmeat Loaf

INGREDIENTS

2 cups	TVP
1 large	onion
2 stalks	celery
2 blade	scallion
2 Tbsp	soy sauce
1 cup	whole wheat or spelt bread crumbs
3 cloves	garlic
1 tsp	sage
1 tsp	rosemary
1 tsp	cumin
2 Tbsp	nutritional yeast
2 Tbsp	peanut oil
1 pinch	cayenne
1 Tbsp	unbleached flour
	salt to taste

DIRECTIONS

1. Soak TVP. Add sage, rosemary, and soy sauce. Let sit for half an hour.
2. Chop scallion, celery, garlic, and onion very fine and sauté.
3. Mix with soaked TVP. Add flour, cumin, nutritional yeast, and bread crumbs.
4. Add salt to taste. Put into small loaf baking pan and bake at 350F for one hour.

Chickpea Loaf

INGREDIENTS

2 cups	chickpeas (soaked for 5 hours or overnight)
1 large	onion
2 blades	celery
3 blades	scallion
2 cloves	garlic
1 tsp	sage
2 Tbsp	chickpea flour or flour of your choice
1 tsp	marjoram
1 tsp	basil
1 tsp	oregano
1 tsp	thyme
1 Tbsp	sesame oil
2 tsp	sea salt
1 tsp	cumin
1 Tbsp	paprika

DIRECTIONS

1. Boil chickpeas and grind in food processor.
2. Sauté the rest of ingredients, except flour.
3. Add ingredients to ground chickpeas and mix until all ingredients have been incorporated.
4. Add flour and sprinkle with paprika.
5. Place in a greased loaf pan at 350F for 45 minutes.

Cauliflower and Broccoli Au Gratin

INGREDIENTS

1 head	cauliflower (cut into florets)
1 head	broccoli (cut into florets)
½ cup	nutritional yeast
1 med	onion, chopped
2 cloves	garlic, chopped
1 pinch	cumin
1 pinch	marjoram
1 pinch	turmeric
1 pinch	dry mustard
½ cup	unbleached flour
1 tsp	sea salt
1 ½ cups	water
2 Tbsp	peanut oil

DIRECTIONS

1. Sauté onion, garlic, cumin, marjoram, sea salt, and turmeric.
2. Add flour to mixture and stir. Add water, nutritional yeast and mustard.
3. Keep stirring until everything is mixed into a thick paste.
4. Steam broccoli and cauliflower. Line 9-inch baking dish with steamed broccoli and cauliflower.
5. Pour on sauce and bake at 350F for 30 minutes.

Vegetable Quiche with Tofu

INGREDIENTS

1 pkg	firm tofu
2 Tbsp	olive oil
1 med	green pepper, diced
1 med	red pepper, diced
1 small	onion
1 pinch	basil
1 pinch	oregano
½ cup	green beans
1 pinch	salt
2 Tbsp	cornstarch
2 cloves	garlic
2 blades	scallion (green onions)
1 cup	fresh mushroom slices
1 cup	yellow squash, diced

DIRECTIONS

1. Blend tofu, salt, cornstarch, basil and oregano until smooth and creamy.

2. Sauté minced garlic, scallions, onion, green and red peppers.

3. Add bended mixture to sautéed vegetables and mix well until completely mixed.

4. Pour into a prepared pie dish and bake for 20 minutes at 375F.

Vegetarian Delight

INGREDIENTS

2 cups	textured protein (TVP) (soaked in warm water)
¼ cup	nutritional yeast
3 cups	warm water
3 blades	green onion
2 blades	fresh thyme
2 cloves	garlic
1 small	onion, diced
1 small	green pepper, diced
1 small	red pepper, diced
1 tsp	sage
1 tsp	cumin
1 tsp	oregano
1 Tbsp	vegetable oil
1 tsp	basil
1 Tbsp	soy sauce
1 Tbsp	cooking oil
4 blades	celery, cut across in 1/4 - inch bits
1 Tbsp	blackstrap molasses
2 Tbsp	tomato paste (optional)

DIRECTIONS

1. Sauté half of above ingredients, except celery in one tablespoon cooking oil. Save remaining seasoning and set aside.

2. Add soaked TVP to sautéed mixture. If dry, add additional cup of water. Salt to taste.

3. Stir in blackstrap molasses, tomato paste, and nutritional yeast. Cook for 15 minutes. Turn off stove.

4. Sauté saved ingredients and soy sauce with celery and one tablespoon of cooking oil for approximately 10 minutes.

5. Add salt to taste and pour over TVP to garnish. Serve over rice.

Tofu Cutlets

INGREDIENTS

1 pkg	**tofu, extra firm**
½ cup	**nutritional yeast**
2 Tbsp	**whole wheat flour or flour of choice**
1 pinch	**Spike seasoning**
2 Tbsp	**poultry seasoning**

DIRECTIONS

1. Rinse and cut tofu into strips 4 inches long. Drain off excess water.
2. Put nutritional yeast, flour, poultry seasoning and Spike into a plastic bag and shake to mix.
3. Put a few strips of tofu into bag and shake.
4. Heat oil and fry, turning the tofu on each side until golden brown.
5. Can be used as a breakfast treat or sandwich filling.

Stewed Vegetable Chunks

INGREDIENTS

1 cup	veggie chunks (soy protein)
2	vegetable bouillon cubes
2 med	potatoes
2 med	carrots
	celery
1 tsp	basil
1 tsp	rosemary
1 tsp	sage
1 stick	cinnamon
5 whole	cloves
1 med	onion
3 cloves	garlic
1 small	fresh ginger piece
	(use a dark sauce to color)
3 cups	water
1 pinch	brown sugar
2 Tbsp	flour
1 Tbsp	vegetable oil
1 pinch	thyme
2 Tbsp	nutritional yeast
	Spike seasoning to taste

DIRECTIONS

1. Heat vegetable oil. Stir in flour. Keep stirring until slightly brown.

2. Add water, cinnamon, clove, ginger, rosemary, and sage.

3. Cut celery, potatoes, and carrots in one-inch bits and add to water along with the vegetable chunks.

4. Let cook for 20 minutes. Add remaining spices to taste and cook for another 10 minutes.

5. Serve with brown rice. Serves four.

Curried Potatoes and Carrots

INGREDIENTS

4 med	potatoes
3 med	carrots
1 med	onion
1 small	piece of ginger
1 tsp	cumin
1 tsp	turmeric
1 Tbsp	curry powder
1 tsp	garam masala
1 Tbsp	vegetable oil
2	bay leaves
1	scotch bonnet pepper
1 pkg	coconut cream or 1 cup freshly prepared coconut milk
1 quart	water
1 tsp	thyme
4 cloves	garlic, diced
	sea salt to taste

DIRECTIONS

1. Sauté, onion, garlic, curry powder and turmeric.
2. Add 1 quart water, coconut cream, carrots, potatoes, remaining seasoning and salt to taste. and bring to boil.
3. Simmer until potatoes and carrots are soft.
4. Add salt to taste if necessary.

Baked Chickette

INGREDIENTS

1 large	Chickette
1 small	onion
2 cloves	garlic
3 blades	scallion
1 pinch	sea salt
1 stalk	celery
1 Tbsp	vegetable oil
½ tsp	basil
1 tsp	soy sauce or molasses
½ tsp	thyme
1/8 tsp	sage
1/8 tsp	oregano
3	pimento grains

DIRECTIONS

1. Cut Chickette into four pieces.
2. Combine all herbs and spices, molasses and blend together in food processor.
3. Add sea salt to blended mixture.
4. Stick the Chickettes with a sharp knife, making holes in them.
5. Stuff seasoning into Chickette and rub some oil on the Chickette.
6. Grease baking pan and place Chickette into pan. Cover with foil.
7. Bake for 30 minutes. Remove foil and bake until it begins to get brown.
8. Turn Chickette until all sides are brown. Serve by slicing.

TVP Vegetable Medley

INGREDIENTS

1 cup	TVP
1 tsp	sage
1 tsp	thyme
2 Tbsp	nutritional yeast
1 tsp	ginger
1 stalk	cilantro
1 stalk	scallion
1 pinch	oregano
1 pinch	basil
1 Tbsp	vegetable oil
1 pinch	whole rosemary
1 cup	string beans
1 cup	carrots
1/2 cup	red pepper
1/2 cup	green pepper
1/2 cup	onion
2 Tbsp	dark mushroom sauce, molasses or tomato paste to color TVP
	sea salt to taste

DIRECTIONS

1. Sauté onion for two minutes.
2. Add TVP and enough water to soften TVP.
3. Cook for 10 minutes then add remaining ingredients.
4. Cook until tender. Add salt to taste and serve.

Cous Cous Medley

INGREDIENTS

1 cup	cous cous
1 blade	scallion
1 small	onion
1 blade	garlic
1 blade	celery
1 Tbsp	margarine
1 pinch	Spike seasoning or seasoning of choice
1 ½ cup	water
1 pinch	basil
1 small	green pepper
1 small	red pepper

DIRECTIONS

1. Chop finely onion, scallion, garlic and celery. Sauté in margarine.

2. Add water, Spike and basil. Boil for 2 minutes.

3. Add cous cous. Water should be a little above cous cous.

4. Stir, cover and turn off fire.

5. Let stand for 2 minutes and fluff with fork and garnish with peppers.

6. Cover for another 2 minutes and serve with a salad.

BBQ Tofu

INGREDIENTS

1 pkg	tofu, firm
1 tsp	poultry seasoning
1 tsp	turmeric
1 pinch	garlic powder
1 tsp	paprika
1 cup	peanut oil
	sea salt to taste

DIRECTIONS

1. Cut tofu in 1-inch bits.
2. Place all ingredients in a plastic bag and shake lightly until all tofu is covered with seasoning.
3. Heat oil and fry tofu until light crust forms.
4. Drain well. Heat your favorite BBQ sauce and pour on tofu.

Three Bean Burger

INGREDIENTS

1 cup	chick peas
1 cup	black beans
1 cup	soybeans or navy beans
1 small	onion
2 cloves	garlic
1 Tbsp	cumin
1 pinch	turmeric
2 Tbsp	wheat flour
1 tsp	Italian seasoning
2 blades	celery
	Spike seasoning to taste

DIRECTIONS

1. Cook three beans separately until soft. Mash beans and combine all in a large bowl.

2. Chop onions, garlic, celery, very small and sauté for 3 minutes.

3. Add this to mashed beans. Add turmeric, cumin, flour, and Spike seasoning to taste.

4. Shape into burgers and dip burgers into flour.

5. Fry in a small amount of oil on both sides.

6. Drain and serve in burger rolls with lettuce and tomatoes.

Vegan Macaroni Uncheese

INGREDIENTS

2 cups	macaroni
1 small	onion, diced
1 cup	diced red pepper
1 cup	diced green pepper
1 cup	diced celery
1 clove	garlic
4 cups	water
1 heaping Tbsp	turmeric
2 cups	milk (soy, almond or rice)
¼ cup	nutritional yeast
	sea salt to taste

DIRECTIONS

1. Boil 8 cups of water, add the macaroni and turmeric and salt. Boil macaroni until tender but not too soft. Drain macaroni and run cold water on it.

2. Sauté remaining ingredients. Add nutritional yeast and milk. Bring to boil. Add cooked macaroni and combine. Serve.

Chickpea Patties

INGREDIENTS

3 cups	chickpeas
1 small	onion
2 cloves	garlic
1 heaping Tbsp	cumin
1 Tbsp	nutritional yeast
1 pinch	turmeric
2 Tbsp	wheat flour
1 tsp	Italian seasoning
2 blades	celery
	sea salt to taste

DIRECTIONS

1. Cook beans until soft. Mash beans and combine all in a large bowl.
2. Chop onions, garlic, celery, very small and sauté for 3 minutes.
3. Add this to mashed beans. Add turmeric, cumin, nutritional yeast and flour.
4. Shape into burgers and dip burgers into flour.
5. Fry in a small amount of oil on both sides.
6. Drain and serve in burger rolls with lettuce and tomatoes.

Vegetable Pie

INGREDIENTS

1 cup	carrot wheels
½ cup	mushrooms thinly sliced
¼ lb	button onions
2 Tbsp	soy margarine
2 cloves	garlic finely diced
1 tsp	agar agar
½ cup	shredded soy cheese
1 tsp	egg replacer
1 sprig	parsley for garnish
1 cup	green beans
2 Tbsp	unbleached flour
1 cup	water
1 Tbsp	Spike seasoning
	sea salt to taste

DIRECTIONS

1. Make pastry and line 9-inch pie dish. Place pie dish in oven and bake for 10 minutes.

2. Sauté onion in soy margarine. Add 1 cup water. Boil for 1 minute.

3. Add remaining ingredients, except flour. Make a thick smooth paste with flour and mix all ingredients together.

4. Pour mixture on baked crust and cover with pastry. Bake for 30 minutes at 350F.

Tofu Stir Fry

INGREDIENTS

1 small	broccoli head
1 small	cauliflower head
1 large	carrot
16 oz	tofu, firm
2 Tbsp	oil
1 small	onion, chopped
1	green pepper, chopped
1	red pepper, chopped
2 cloves	garlic, chopped
2 Tbsp	tamari sauce
	Spike seasoning
1 piece	ginger, finely chopped

DIRECTIONS

1. Cut tofu in 1-inch bits. Soak tofu in soy sauce and a pinch of Spike seasoning for an hour.

2. Heat oil. Sauté tofu without breaking it up. Drain, and place in a bowl.

3. Sauté onion, ginger garlic, and peppers in a little oil.

4. Cut broccoli and cauliflower into florets and cut carrots into 2-inch thin strips and add to seasoning.

5. Cover and cook for 5 minutes. Stir occasionally. Add tofu and serve.

Vegetable Lo Mein

(An easy and relaxing alternative to stir frying)

INGREDIENTS

1 pkg	linguine or spaghetti
1 Tbsp	oriental sesame oil
2 Tbsp	tamari soy sauce
¼ cup	peanut oil
3 sprigs	fresh thyme, stripped
3 stalks	celery
2 cups	string beans, 2 inches in length
3 med	carrots, cut in 2-inch thin strips
½ small	cabbage, cut in strips
1 med	onion
1 pkg	extra firm tofu cut in 1-inch cubes, seasoned to taste with tamari sauce and patted dry
2 cloves	garlic, minced
1 Tbsp	fresh ginger
4 ½ cups	thinly sliced mushrooms
2	scallions, thinly sliced

DIRECTIONS

1. Cook the pasta in a large pot of boiling water. The pasta should be a little chewy in texture.

2. Drain very well in a colander. Mix sesame oil and soy sauce together then pour over pasta and toss to coat.

3. Place in a baking dish and cover. Keep warm at 300F in oven while stir-frying vegetables.

4. In a wok or large skillet, heat 2 tablespoons of the peanut oil over high heat until hot but not smoking.

5. Add tofu and stir until golden all over. Drain and remove to a platter.

6. Reduce heat to medium and add the remaining peanut oil along with remaining ingredients: garlic, onion, ginger, mushrooms, scallions, cabbage, carrots, string beans, celery, and fresh thyme.

7. Stir fry the garlic and ginger for 30 seconds. Add mushrooms and stir fry until brown and juicy, about 7 minutes.

8. Return tofu to pan and toss. Add the scallions and stir fry 2 minutes.

9. Sprinkle on the soy sauce and sesame oil and toss again.

10. Remove the pasta from oven and add sautéed vegetables and tofu. Toss thoroughly and add soy sauce to taste.

11. Serve immediately or cover and keep warm in the oven for up to 20 minutes. Serves 3 to 4.

Coconut Curry Vegetables

Coconut milk flavored with curry makes a rich and luscious sauce for carrots, acorn squash, kombucha squash and broccoli. Scotch bonnet peppers make it fiery. Serve with a nutty brown rice such as Basmati.

INGREDIENTS

2 Tbsp	peanut oil
3 large	garlic cloves minced
1 med	yellow onion sliced or chopped
2 large	carrots sliced ¼ -inch thick on the diagonal
½ med	acorn, butternut, or kombucha squash (cut in bite-size pieces)
3 Tbsp	curry powder
14 oz	coconut milk
1	scotch bonnet pepper
2 cups	broccoli florets
2 cups	cauliflower
2 cups	chickpeas (cooked)
1 Tbsp	cumin
1 tsp	garam masala
1 Tbsp	tamari sauce
	sea salt to taste

DIRECTIONS

1. Heat the oil in a large heavy pot. Add garlic and onions.

2. Cook over high heat for 2 to 4 minutes, stirring frequently. When the onions begin to look translucent, toss in squash and carrots.

3. Cook for a few minutes to sauté the vegetables then stir in curry powder.

4. Reduce heat to medium. Continue to cook for 5 minutes. If vegetables begin to stick to pan, add ¼ cup water.

5. Stir in coconut milk and scotch bonnet pepper, partially cover and simmer for about 30 minutes or until vegetables are tender. The coconut milk will cook down to a stew-like consistency. Add a little water if you need more sauce.

6. When the vegetables are soft, stir in broccoli and simmer for 5 minutes until broccoli turns a bright green and is still crunchy.

7. Stir in chickpeas and season with cumin and pepper to taste. Add salt to taste. Remove from heat.

Brown Rice and Peas

INGREDIENTS

2 cups	brown rice
1 cup	red peas
6 oz	coconut cream
2 cloves	garlic, chopped
1 small	onion, chopped
1 pinch	brown sugar
3 sprigs	fresh thyme
1 bundle	scallions
6 cups	water
	salt to taste

DIRECTIONS

1. Pick and wash peas and rice. Keep separate.
2. Boil peas in 6 cups of water. Add coconut cream and a little garlic, onion and thyme.
3. Boil for 30 minutes. Add brown rice, salt, sugar and rest of seasonings.
4. Cook in a tightly sealed pot for best results. Lower fire and simmer until rice absorbs all water. Add more water if necessary.
5. Stir one time with a large fork.

Princess's Yellow Rice

INGREDIENTS

2 cups	brown rice
1 heaping tsp	turmeric
1 small	onion
3 cloves	garlic
pinch	sage
pinch	rosemary
2 sprigs	scallion
1	red pepper
1	green pepper, diced
1 large	carrot, diced
8 cups	filtered water
	salt to taste

DIRECTIONS

1. Bring water to boil. Add turmeric and rice.
2. Cook rice for 10 to 15 minutes until rice grains swell but are not very soft.
3. Take rice off fire and wash with cold water. Drain in colander for 5 minutes.
4. Sauté the rest of ingredients together including salt.
5. Add rice and keep stirring for 6 minutes.
6. Shut off stove and serve.

Spicy Squash Stew

INGREDIENTS

¾ cup	almonds
½ cup	sesame seeds
¼ Tbsp	peanut oil
3 large	garlic cloves, minced
1	yellow onion chopped
1 med	butternut squash (about 2 lbs cut in 1-inch bits)
2 ½ cups	sliced mushrooms
1 ½ tsp	dried oregano
¼ tsp	chili powder
1 tsp	crushed red pepper flakes
1 cup	chopped tomatoes
½ cup	water
2 cups	cauliflower florets
2 cups	fresh or frozen green peas
2 Tbsp	tamari
	pepper to taste

DIRECTIONS

1. In a dry skillet, toast almonds over medium heat for 5 minutes until slightly brown.

2. Set aside and use same pot to roast sesame seeds. Keep tossing pan to prevent them from burning.

3. In a food processor grind the almonds and sesame seeds to coarse powder.

4. Heat the oil in a heavy pot or wok. Sauté onion, garlic over medium heat for 3 to 4 minutes, stirring frequently.

5. When the onions are translucent, stir in squash, mushroom, cumin, oregano, chili powder and pepper.

6. Continue cooking over medium heat for 5 minutes. If the vegetables begin to stick to pan, add one tablespoon of water.

7. Add tomatoes and enough water to cover all vegetables. Partially cover and simmer until squash is soft, about 10 minutes.

8. Check to make sure enough liquid is covering vegetables. If not, add more water to cover.

9. When squash is soft, add almonds, sesame seeds and cauliflower.

10. Simmer for 10 minutes then add peas. Cook for one minute.

11. Season with tamari and pepper. Serve.

PART 3
Super Soups and Stews

- Split Pea Soup
- Pumpkin Soup
- Veggie Jamaican Pepper Pot Soup
- Black Bean Soup
- Cream of Broccoli Soup
- Cream of Pumpkin
- Vegetable Barley Soup

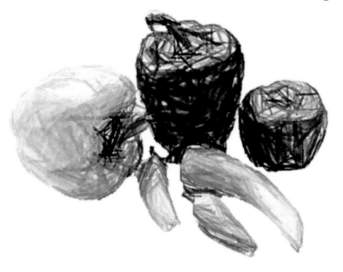

Split Pea Soup

INGREDIENTS

2 cups	dried split peas, green or yellow
2 quarts	water
2	tomatoes, chopped
1 small	onion, chopped
1 cup	pumpkin, acorn or black forest squash
1 blade	celery, chopped
2 cloves	garlic, chopped
½ tsp	cilantro
3 blades	scallion
1 Tbsp	olive oil
1 large	carrot
1 large	potato cut in small pieces
	Spike seasoning to taste

DIRECTIONS

1. Cook split peas until they start to open up.
2. Add onions, carrots, potatoes, tomatoes, cilantro, celery and pumpkin.
3. Cook for 20 minutes. Then add remaining spices and cook for another 15 minutes.
4. Add olive oil and serve.

Pumpkin Soup

INGREDIENTS

3 quarts	water
3 heaping Tbsp	barley
1 cup	pumpkin
3 med	Irish potatoes
1 large	carrot
1 med	onion
2 blades	scallions
1 inch piece	fresh ginger
2 ripe	tomatoes
3 stalks	celery
1 pinch	cayenne pepper
2	bay leaves
7	pimento grains
1 pinch	marjoram
½ stick	margarine
1 cup	fresh coconut milk (optional)
	salt to taste

DIRECTIONS

1. Bring water to a boil.
2. Wash and cut carrots, potatoes, and pumpkin into 1-inch bits.
3. Add to water along with barley and ginger. Cook until barley is tender.
4. Add rest of ingredients and cook for 10 minutes. Serve hot.

Veggie Jamaican Pepper Pot Soup

INGREDIENTS

2 lbs	spinach, cut fine
1 dozen	okras cut in small rings
1 lb	coco or Irish potatoes
1 whole	unbroken green hot pepper (optional)
1 med	onion, chopped
1 clove	garlic, crushed
1	zucchini
1 small	eggplant, chopped coarsely
1 ½ lbs	kale, chopped fine
3 blades	scallion, chopped fine
2 sprigs	thyme
1 quart	water
2 Tbsp	virgin or cold-pressed olive oil
1 cup	coconut milk or ½ pkg cream of coconut
6	pimento seeds
3	bay leaves
	sea salt to taste

DIRECTIONS

1. Boil water. Add coco, bay leaves, pimento seeds, and coconut milk.
2. Steam spinach and kale in another saucepan and blend.
3. Add to pot eggplant, okra, zucchini and hot peppers.
4. Sauté garlic, onion, scallion, thyme, coconut milk and sea salt to taste.
5. Add these ingredients when soup has been boiled for 30 minutes and simmer for another 5 minutes.

Black Bean Soup

INGREDIENTS

2 cups	black beans
2 stalks or leaves	cilantro
1 tsp	sea salt
1 small	onion
2 blades	scallion
2 cloves	garlic
1 stalk	celery
1 tsp	thyme, fresh or dried
½ tsp	sage
½ tsp	rosemary
4 cups	water
2	bay leaves
1 cup	coconut milk

DIRECTIONS

1. Soak beans overnight before cooking and discard soaking water.
2. Cook black beans in water, coconut milk and add bay leaves. Cook until soft.
3. Sauté all seasonings and add to beans. Boil for 10 minutes.
4. Shut off stove. Let stand for 5 minutes and serve.

Cream of Broccoli Soup

INGREDIENTS

1 bundle	broccoli
4 cups	soy milk
2 Tbsp	fresh basil
1 pinch	sage
1 pinch	rosemary
3 Tbsp	whole wheat flour
¼ tsp	nutmeg
1/8 tsp	sea salt
1/8 tsp	cayenne pepper
2 cloves	garlic
1 small	onion
1 cup	distilled water

DIRECTIONS

1. Bring water to a boil in saucepan.
2. Add broccoli and cook for 5 minutes.
3. Sauté onion, garlic, basil, flour, rosemary, sage and nutmeg for one minute.
4. Add milk and keep stirring.
5. Blend broccoli in food processor. Blend for 1 minute.
6. Return mixture to saucepan and cook for 5 minutes.
7. Add cayenne and salt taste.

Cream of Pumpkin Soup

INGREDIENTS

1 cup	pumpkin
2 cups	water
2 blades	celery
2 blades	scallions
1 sprig	thyme
1 cup	soy milk
2 Tbsp	unbleached flour
2 cloves	garlic
1 small	onion
1 Tbsp	soy margarine
	salt to taste

DIRECTIONS

1. Boil pumpkin with half of celery, thyme, onion, and garlic until pumpkin is soft. Strain and blend.
2. Return to stove and bring to a boil.
3. Add soy milk and rest of seasonings.
4. Make a paste with unbleached flour and add to soup.
5. Cook for 15 minutes.

Vegetable Barley Soup

INGREDIENTS

1 cup	onion
1 cup	carrots, diced
1 cup	barley, uncooked
2 stalks	celery
2 sprigs	fresh thyme
1 cup	turnips diced
1 cup	diced Caribbean sweet potato
1 cup	green beans
½ tsp	marjoram
8 ½ cups	filtered water
2 Tbsp	parsley
1 cube	vegetable bouillon or I ½ Tbsp nutritional yeast (optional)
	salt to taste

DIRECTIONS

1. Place water in a pot. Add barley and cook for ten minutes.

2. Add carrots and all other ingredients except onion, garlic, thyme, and parsley. Cook for 40 minutes.

3. Add remaining seasonings except parsley. Garnish with parsley.

PART 4
Sassy Salads, Sensational Sauces & Salad Dressings

- Crunchy Lentil Salad
- Tabouli
- Blueberry Sauce
- Hummus (Chickpea Paste)
- Sweet and Sour Sauce
- Tomato Sauce
- Plum Sauce
- Strawberry Rhubarb Sauce
- Cashew Ginger Sauce
- Parsley Tahini Dressing
- Ranch Dressing
- Lemon Salad Dressing
- French Dressing
- Avocado Dressing
- Supreme Salad Dressing

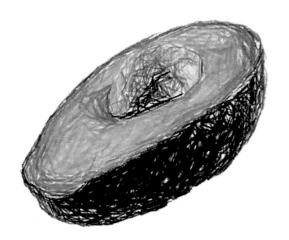

Crunchy Lentil Salad

INGREDIENTS

1 cup	lentils, picked over and rinsed
5 cups	water
1	bay leaf
1	carrot, minced
1	celery rib, finely diced
¼ cup	onion, finely diced
2 Tbsp	fresh parsley, minced
¼ cup	fruity olive oil (Spanish extra virgin)
2 Tbsp	freshly squeezed lemon juice
1	garlic clove, pressed or minced
¼ tsp	dried thyme
¼ tsp	ground cumin

DIRECTIONS

1. In medium saucepan combine lentils, water and bay leaves.

2. Bring to a boil and cook uncovered for 15 minutes or until lentils are tender but still crunchy. Stir occasionally.

3. Pour into a colander and discard bay leaves. Drain lentils very well and let sit for 5 minutes.

4. Make sure water is completely drained. Place the lentils in a serving bowl and gently stir in celery, carrots, onion and parsley.

5. Mix together olive oil, lemon juice, garlic, thyme, cumin, salt and pepper. Pour into the lentil mixture and carefully toss.

6. Use salt, pepper or Braggs Amino Acids to taste. Serve at room temperature.

7. (Keeping the lentils slightly crunchy and dressing them with a small amount of olive oil, lemon juice, and spices contributes to this salad's light consistency. Can be served alongside a baked potato for a quick complete meal. Serves 4 as a main course.)

Tabouli

INGREDIENTS

2	plum tomatoes (diced)
1 med	zucchini (diced)
½ cup	cooked chickpeas
1 cup	bulgar wheat
2 Tbsp	olive oil
1 tsp	fresh mint
1	lemon juice
1 pinch	seasoning salt
1 ½ cup	water, Shoshu, Tamari or Braggs Liquid Aminos sauce

DIRECTIONS

1. Soak bulgar wheat in warm water until it swells and softens.
2. Add remaining ingredients, marinate and place in refrigerator.

Blueberry Sauce

INGREDIENTS

3 Tbsp   sugar or honey
2 cups   fresh blueberries
2 Tbsp   lemon juice
1/3 cup   water

DIRECTIONS

1. Combine all ingredients and cook over medium heat.

2. Stir until mixture is thickened.

3. Serve warm or cold over pancakes.

Hummus (Chickpea Paste)

INGREDIENTS

1 ½ cup	chickpeas (garbanzo beans)
3 quarts	water
¼ cup	sesame tahini
3 Tbsp	lemon juice
2 cloves	garlic
1 pinch	salt

DIRECTIONS

1. Soak garbanzo beans overnight. Throw off water beans were soaked in. Bring 3 quarts water to a boil and boil beans until tender. Drain off water and let cool.

2. Grind beans in food processor with tahini, garlic, lemon juice and pinch of salt to taste.

Sweet and Sour Sauce

INGREDIENTS

1 cup	brown sugar
½ cup	apple cider vinegar
2 Tbsp	soy sauce
2 Tbsp	Sherry
3 Tbsp	tomato sauce
2 Tbsp	cornstarch
½ cup	pineapple juice

DIRECTIONS

1. Combine sugar, vinegar, soy sauce, and sherry to make sauce.
2. Bring to a boil then add cornstarch and pineapple juice.
3. Stir until sauce is thickened.

Tomato Sauce

INGREDIENTS

2 ½ cups	fresh plum tomatoes, chopped
3 cloves	garlic minced
2 Tbsp	olive oil
2 Tbsp	tomato paste
½ tsp	sea salt
2 tsp	dried basil or fresh
½ tsp	cayenne pepper (optional)

DIRECTIONS

1. Sauté garlic in olive oil until barely tan.
2. Add remaining ingredients, except pepper and cook uncovered for 30 minutes or until the sauce is fairly thick.
3. Add pepper mix. Cover pot and turn off stove.
4. Let cool for a little and serve with rice or mashed potatoes.

Plum Sauce

INGREDIENTS

10	fresh plums
¼ cup	dried apricots soaked in warm water
1 tsp	chili sauce
1 tsp	salt
2 Tbsp	water
½ cup	vinegar

DIRECTIONS

1. Place plums and apricots in wok. Add chili sauce, salt and water.

2. Bring to boil and simmer gently for 15 minutes.

3. Add a little more water if the mixture becomes too dry.

4. Stir in sugar and simmer 20 to 30 minutes until sauce reaches chutney-like consistency.

5. Pour sauce into a sterilized bottle.

Strawberry Rhubarb Sauce

INGREDIENTS

1 quart   **strawberries**
10 stalks   **rhubarb, sliced diagonally a third of an inch**
          thick
          maple syrup

DIRECTIONS

1. Wash strawberries and rhubarb.
2. Hull strawberries with a sharp paring knife and thickly slice them.
3. Place the fruit in a pot with half a cup of water and simmer until everything is pink (about 20 minutes).
4. Add maple syrup to taste.
5. Serve with yogurt for breakfast or with ice cream for a late night snack.

Cashew Ginger Sauce

INGREDIENTS

1 cup	cashew
3 inches	ginger
¼ cup	peanut oil
2 med	garlic cloves, minced
2 Tbsp	tamari
1 Tbsp	fresh cilantro, chopped
1	lime, juiced
¾ cup	hot water

DIRECTIONS

1. In dry skillet, toast cashews over medium heat for 5 minutes, tossing continually to prevent burning.

2. Peel and grate ginger in a towel or hand-squeeze juice from ginger into a food processor.

3. Add all ingredients except water in food processor and blend until smooth and creamy.

4. Continue to blend, adding the water a little at a time.

5. The zesty flavor of ginger and lime balance the sweetness of the cashews.

6. This sauce goes well with hot steamed vegetables or tossed fettuccine. It is also an excellent substitute for sour cream in stroganoffs.

Parsley Tahini Dressing

INGREDIENTS

½ cup	spring water
1 pinch	onion powder
1	lemon, juiced
½ cup	sesame butter
1 clove	garlic
4 blades	fresh parsley
1 pinch	cayenne (optional)
	cumin to taste
	sea salt to taste

DIRECTIONS

1. Blend all ingredients.

Ranch Dressing

INGREDIENTS

1 cup	tofu
½ cup	soy milk
½ cup	Nasoya mayonnaise
2 Tbsp	scallions
2 Tbsp	fresh parsley
1 tsp	prepared mustard
¼ tsp	garlic
¼ tsp	onion powder
1 pinch	dill
1 pinch	cayenne pepper

DIRECTIONS

1. Blend all ingredients and chill several hours before serving. Makes 2 ½ cups.

Lemon Salad Dressing

INGREDIENTS

¾ cup   **vegetable or olive oil**
½ cup   **lemon juice**
1 ½ Tbsp   **honey**
½ tsp   **tarragon**
½ tsp   **thyme**
¼ tsp   **pepper**
1 clove   **garlic, crushed**

DIRECTIONS

1. Combine all ingredients and shake well. Chill overnight.

French Dressing

INGREDIENTS

¾ cup	cold pressed Olive oil
½ cup	lemon juice
1 small	onion
¼ tsp	parsley
1 pinch	cumin
1 pinch	brown sugar
8 plum	tomatoes (or 2 large beefy tomatoes)
¼ tsp	oregano
¼ tsp	basil
	salt to taste

DIRECTIONS

1. Blend all ingredients while slowly adding olive oil. Taste for flavor.

Avocado Dressing

INGREDIENTS

1 large	avocado (ripe)
1 tsp	sea salt
1 Tbsp	olive oil
2 cloves	garlic
¼ tsp	mustard seed oil
¼ tsp	cayenne pepper
1 Tbsp	honey
1	onion

DIRECTIONS

1. Scoop out avocado flesh and place in blender. Add other ingredients and blend.

Supreme Salad Dressing

INGREDIENTS

2 Tbsp	chickpea miso
2 Tbsp	sesame tahini
2 large	dates (pitted)
2	mint leaves
2 Tbsp	lemon juice
½ cup	filtered water
2 Tbsp	carrots

DIRECTIONS

1. Blend all ingredients and serve with salad.

PART 5
Tasty Drinks

- Energy Drink
- Almond Milk
- Banana Soy and Maple Shake
- Energy Shake
- Apple Lemon Cooler
- Banana Peanut Punch
- Breadfruit Drink

Energy Drink

INGREDIENTS

1 Tbsp	almond nuts
1 Tbsp	sunflower seeds
1 Tbsp	pumpkin seeds
1 cup	spring or filtered water
1 pinch	nutmeg
1 pinch	cinnamon
3 drops	vanilla extract
	sweetener of choice

DIRECTIONS

1. Soak all nuts and seeds a few hours before making drink.
2. Blend the seeds and nuts with water and add the remaining ingredients.
3. Sweeten with brown sugar, honey, maple syrup or any sweetener of your choice.

Almond Milk

INGREDIENTS

1 cup	filtered or spring water
¼ cup	almond nuts
¼ tsp	vanilla extract
¼ tsp	almond extract
1 Tbsp	sunflower seeds

DIRECTIONS

1. Soak almonds overnight. Drain and rinse.
2. Blend almonds until creamy.
3. Strain through cheese cloth.
4. Sweeten with your favorite sweetener and serve.

Banana Soy and Maple Shake

INGREDIENTS

1 ripe	banana (speckled banana)
1 cup	soy milk
1 tsp	lecithin
2 tsp	wheat germ
2 tsp	maple syrup or honey
1 tsp	fresh lemon juice

DIRECTIONS

1. Combine all ingredients in blender.
2. Puree until smooth and frothy.

Energy Shake

INGREDIENTS

2 Tbsp	parsley (fresh)
6	carrots

DIRECTIONS

1. Juice and drink.

Apple Lemon Cooler

INGREDIENTS

6	apples
1	lemon

DIRECTIONS

1. Juice apples and lemon. Combine and serve. Garnish with a slice of lemon.

Banana Peanut Punch

INGREDIENTS

2 or 3 ripe	bananas
3 cups	soy milk
1 tsp	vanilla extract
2 heaping Tbsp	peanut butter

DIRECTIONS

1. Blend all ingredients until creamy.
2. Sweeten with your favorite sweetener and serve.

Breadfruit Drink

INGREDIENTS

2 cups	boiled, ripe breadfruit
1 large	coconut (dry)
1 pinch	cinnamon
1 pinch	vanilla
1 pinch	freshly grated nutmeg
1 pinch	sea salt (optional)
1 cup	water
	sugar, maple syrup or honey to taste

DIRECTIONS

1. Wash coconut meat and blend with approximately 4 cups of water. Strain coconut milk.

2. Divide breadfruit in half. Blend half of all ingredients and pour into mug. Blend the remaining half.

3. Mix all in mug, chill and serve.

PART 6
Delectable Desserts

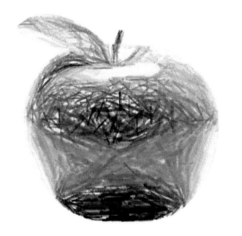

- Carrot Cake
- Date Nut Bread
- Easter Spice Bun
- Coconut Buns
- Cartwheel Cookies
- Coconut Delight
- Banana Nut Bread
- Fresh Plum Tart
- Apple Pie
- Apple Crum Pie
- Hot Cross Buns
- Pumpkin Tea Bread
- Whole Wheat Fruit Muffins
- Pie Crust

Carrot Cake

INGREDIENTS

2 cups	carrot pulp
½ cup	vegetable oil
2 cups	brown sugar
¾ cups	walnuts
2 Tbsp	egg replacer
2 tsp	cinnamon
1 tsp	nutmeg
3 cups	whole wheat flour
2 ½ tsp	baking powder
1 tsp	baking soda
1 1/3 cup	soy milk
1 cup	filtered water
1 tsp	almond extract
1 tsp	vanilla extract
1 dash	salt

DIRECTIONS

1. Mix oil, sugar and carrot pulp until smooth.
2. Gradually add walnuts, nutmeg and cinnamon.
3. Mix baking soda, baking powder and sea salt into flour and add gradually to above ingredients.
4. Add soy milk, vanilla, almond extract and 1 cup water.
5. Mix egg replacer and one tablespoon water into thick paste and add to mixture. (One teaspoon egg replacer mixed into one tablespoon water is equivalent to two eggs. If mixture is too dry, add additional water to all cake and bread recipes.)
6. Bake for 1 hour at 360F.

Date Nut Bread

INGREDIENTS

1 cup	dates, pitted and chopped
1 tsp	baking soda
1 cup	boiling water
1 Tbsp	soy margarine
2 tsp	egg replacer
2/3 cup	brown sugar
1 tsp	vanilla extract
2 tsp	baking powder
¼ tsp	salt
1 ¾ cup	unsifted whole/wheat flour
1 cup	walnuts, chopped

DIRECTIONS

1. Place chopped pitted dates in a mixing bowl.
2. Sprinkle with baking soda and pour in boiling water.
3. Add margarine and mix.
4. In a second bowl, whisk the egg replacer in a little water until light.
5. Add sugar and vanilla, then baking powder and salt.
6. Blend into the first mixture and mix well.
7. Blend in flour completely and fold in chopped nuts.
8. Pour into a greased 9x5x3 inch loaf pan and bake in a preheated 350F oven for 1 hour until loaf test done.
9. Turn loaf out on rack to cool. When thoroughly cooled, wrap well to store.

Easter Spiced Bun

INGREDIENTS

½ oz	dry yeast
1 whole	nutmeg, grated
1 stick	soy milk
½ lb	soy margarine
1 ½ cup	brown sugar
4 cups	unbleached flour
1 cup	tepid water
1 tsp	egg replacer
1 tsp	sea salt
¼ cup	crystallized, chopped cherries or cranberries
¼ cup	raisins
¼ cup	mix peel (orange, grapefruit, lemon), finely chopped
¼ cup	blackstrap molasses
1 tsp	cinnamon
1 pinch	mix spice

DIRECTIONS

1. Dissolve yeast in small amount of lukewarm water.
2. Heat soy milk and boil the cup of water. Combine liquids.
3. Place butter sugar salt and spice in a bowl and pour in milk and water.
4. Beat egg replacer in tablespoon of milk mixture and add to liquid mixture.
5. Sieve half the flour into the liquid and stir well, then stir in yeast and all fruits.
6. Add sufficient amount of remaining flour to make a stiff dough.
7. Cover and let rise to double in bulk.
8. Knead, then sprinkle in rest of flour and again knead well.
9. Shape into loaves and let rise again until double in bulk.
10. Bake in greased loaf tins at 350F until bun leaves sides of pan and springs to touch.

11. Brush with honey to glaze.

Coconut Buns

INGREDIENTS

2 cups	unbleached flour
2 Tbsp	soy margarine
¼ cup	grated coconut
½ cup	sugar
1 tsp	cinnamon
1 tsp	vanilla
1 tsp	nutmeg
1 tsp	egg replacer
1 Tbsp	baking powder
¼	soy milk or coconut milk

DIRECTIONS

1. Grease baking sheet.
2. Sieve the flour and baking powder together.
3. Cream margarine and sugar.
4. Beat egg replacer in 1 tablespoon of soy milk or coconut milk and add to flour to make a stiff mixture.
5. Stir in coconut and rest of ingredients.
6. Place in small heaps on greased baking sheet.
7. Bake in a heated oven at 375F for 15 to 18 minutes.

Cartwheel Cookies

INGREDIENTS

1 ½ cups	**whole wheat flour**
1 ½ cups	**unbleached flour**
1 tsp	**baking powder**
½ tsp	**aluminum-free baking soda**
¼ tsp	**sea salt**
1 tsp	**cinnamon**
¼ tsp	**nutmeg**
½ tsp	**ground ginger**
½ tsp	**allspice**
1 cup	**brown sugar**
3 Tbsp	**molasses**
2 Tbsp	**melted soy margarine**
One 8 oz glass	**"wet" sugar (sugar with enough added water to make a thick syrup)**

DIRECTIONS

1. Sieve all dry ingredients together.
2. Make a well in center and pour the thick syrup sugar into well.
3. Add melted margarine and blend all together lightly.
4. Turn out onto well-floured board and pat with your hand to a thickness of ¼ - inch or a bit thicker.
5. Cut into circles using an ordinary drinking glass for this purpose.
6. Raise cookies with a well-floured spatula and place on a slightly greased and well-floured cookie sheet.
7. Bake at 400F for 20 minutes.
   **A substitute for "wet" sugar can be made by using 2 ounces of very dark brown sugar and proceeding with sufficient water to make a thick syrup. Add the 3 tablespoons of molasses.

Coconut Delight Cake

INGREDIENTS

2 cups	unbleached flour
1 cup	brown sugar
1 stick	soy margarine
½ cup	soy milk
1 cup	water
2 tsp	baking powder
2 Tbsp	Barbados molasses
2 cups	grated coconut
2 tsp	vanilla
1 tsp	cinnamon
¼ tsp	nutmeg
1 pinch	mixed spice

DIRECTIONS

1. Cream margarine and sugar.
2. Sieve together flour, baking powder, cinnamon, nutmeg and mixed spices.
3. Add soy milk, water and vanilla to above mixture and stir to a stiff paste.
4. Spread evenly in greased shallow baking pan.
5. Bake at 400F for 30 minutes.

Banana Nut Bread

INGREDIENTS

2 cups	unbleached flour
1 tsp	egg replacer
½ cup	brown sugar, honey or maple syrup
2 tsp	baking powder
1 tsp	baking soda
1 tsp	cinnamon
¼ tsp	nutmeg
1 cup	margarine (soy)
½ cup	soy milk
¼ cup	raisins
2 med	bananas, very ripe and crushed
2 tsp	vanilla extract
1 pinch	sea salt
1 cup	margarine

DIRECTIONS

1. Cream margarine and sugar.
2. Mix 3 teaspoon soy milk with one teaspoon egg replacer. Beat well.
3. Add to margarine and sugar. Add crushed banana and mix all together.
4. Add baking powder, cinnamon, nutmeg and salt to flour and mix.
5. Mix in milk and vanilla extract. Add raisins and nuts.
6. Pour into greased loaf pan and bake at 350F for 1 hour or until bread is done when tested.

Fresh Plum Tart

INGREDIENTS

8 med	plums (purple)
1/3 cup	soy margarine
1/3 cup	brown sugar
¼ tsp	vanilla extract
¾ cup	unbleached flour
¼ cup	ground almonds
1 Tbsp	softened margarine
2 ½ Tbsp	brown sugar
1 Tbsp	flour
1 tsp	egg replacer
2 Tbsp	water
1 dash	sea salt

DIRECTIONS

1. Wash and halve the plums in a small mixing bowl.
2. Cream 1/3 cup margarine and sugar until light and fluffy.
3. Mix egg replacer in 1 tablespoon of water and add to margarine and sugar mixture.
4. Beat in vanilla and almond extract.
5. Stir in 3/4 cup flour, 1 Tbsp water, and sea salt.
6. Spread batter evenly over the bottom of a 9" tart pan with removable bottom.
7. Arrange plums, cut side down, over the dough.
8. Sprinkle with 1 ½ tablespoons sugar.
9. Bake in a preheated oven 375F for 30 minutes.
10. Meanwhile, mix almonds with soft margarine, brown sugar and flour.
11. Sprinkle over tart after it has been baked for 30 minutes.
12. Continue to bake 10 to 15 minutes more until crust is golden and plums are tender.

13. Cool on rack. Remove sides of pan and serve warm.

Apple Pie

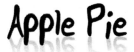

INGREDIENTS

6	apples, cored and sliced (6 cups)
¾ to 1 cup	sugar
2 Tbsp	unbleached flour
½ to 1 tsp	ground cinnamon
2 Tbsp	vegetable margarine
1 dash	ground nutmeg
1 dash	sea salt
Two	9-inch pie shells

DIRECTIONS

1. Combine sugar, unbleached flour, spices and dash of salt. Mix with apples.
2. Fill pie crust with apple mixture. (See Pie Crust recipe on page 116.)
3. Dot with margarine. Cover with pastry.
4. Cut slots in top of crust to allow steam to escape.
5. Sprinkle with sugar. Bake at 400F for 30 minutes or until done.

Apple Crumb Pie

INGREDIENTS

3	Granny Smith apples
½ cup	brown sugar
6 Tbsp	margarine
½ cup	brown sugar
¾ tsp	ground cinnamon
¾ cup	unbleached flour
¼ inch	unbaked 9-inch pastry shell

DIRECTIONS

1. Pare apples, core and cut in eighths.
2. Arrange in unbaked shell. Mix half a cup brown sugar with unbleached flour.
3. Cut in margarine until crumbly. Sprinkle over apples.
4. Bake at 400F for 35 minutes or until done.
5. If pie browns too quickly, cover edge with foil and cool.

Hot Cross Buns

INGREDIENTS

4 cups	**flour**
1 pkg	**dry yeast**
½ tsp	**salt**
2 ozs	**sugar**
1 tsp	**ginger**
2 ozs	**margarine**
1 oz	**mixed peel**
2 ozs	**raisins**
1 cup	**milk**

DIRECTIONS

1. Dissolve yeast in a small amount of lukewarm milk.
2. Let sit for 5 to 10 minutes. Sift dry ingredients together (salt, spice, ginger).
3. Add sugar. Rub into flour.
4. Add warm milk to yeast. Mix in dry ingredients gradually.
5. Knead and sprinkle in raisins.
6. Knead again and allow to rise until double in bulk.
7. Knead once more and shape into loaves or buns.
8. Before baking, make a cross in each bun. Gashes may be filled with honey.
9. Bake at 350F for 35 to 50 minutes.

Pumpkin Tea Bread

This is not too sweet or spicy a bread. It is ideal for serving with mid-morning coffee or afternoon tea. It can be eaten as is or spread with butter. Keeps well in an airtight container.

INGREDIENTS

2 ½ cups	self-rising flour
½ tsp	baking soda
½ tsp	ground cinnamon
½ tsp	freshly grated nutmeg
½ tsp	ground Allspice
½ cup	butter cut into bits (1 stick)
2 Tbsp	maple syrup or honey
1 cup	pumpkin puree
1 cup	soy milk

DIRECTIONS

1. Preheat oven to 375F. Grease 9x5 loaf pan.

2. In large bowl, stir together flour baking soda and spices.

3. Cut in butter until mixture resembles cornmeal.

4. Stir together milk, maple syrup, pumpkin puree and add to flour mix.

5. Beat with a spoon until all ingredients are incorporated, but for as short a time as possible.

6. Place in prepared pan and bake for 50 minutes to 1 hour or until the loaf is well-risen, browned and a toothpick inserted into center comes out clean.

7. Transfer to wire rack and let cool for 30 minutes then take out of the pan and cool completely on rack.

Whole Wheat Fruit Muffins

This is a basic muffin recipe. For variation add chopped fresh fruit, nuts, poppy seeds, or dried cranberries. You can make banana walnut muffins, apple muffins, cranberry banana muffins and so on. Fresh fruits can be substituted with your favorite jam. Fill muffin cups half full with batter, add a teaspoon of jam, and cover with rest of batter. These muffins are quick and fun to make. They taste delectable and the smell is wonderful! Makes 12 small muffins.

INGREDIENTS

2 cups	whole wheat flour
2 Tbsp	baking powder
½ tsp	salt
2/3 cup	honey
½ cup	soft tofu
2 Tbsp	peanut oil
1 ½ cups	soy milk
1 cup	fresh fruit, finely chopped
1 tsp	vanilla
1 tsp	almond extract
½ cup	nuts

DIRECTIONS

1. Preheat oven to 350F.
2. Sift dry ingredients together.
3. In large mixing bowl whisk tofu, oil, honey and milk. Stir in flour.
4. Don't over stir the batter or the muffins will lose their lightness.
5. Stir in chopped fruit or half a cup of nuts.
6. Ladle the batter into well-oiled muffin tins.
7. Bake in the oven for 30 minutes or until top is brown.

Pie Crust

INGREDIENTS

1 cup	whole wheat pastry flour
1 pinch	sea salt
4 oz	soy margarine
	ice water to moisten

DIRECTIONS

1. Mix whole wheat flour and soy margarine with a fork until it looks like fine crumbs.

2. Add small amount of ice water and press flour together into ball.

3. Flatten and roll out about one inch larger than the pie pan.

4. Place dough into pan. Trim and form flattened edge.

5. Bake at 350F for 5 to 10 minutes.

PART 7
Fun Finger Foods

- Bite-Size Vegetable Patties
- Vegetable Fritters
- Ja Coco Fritters

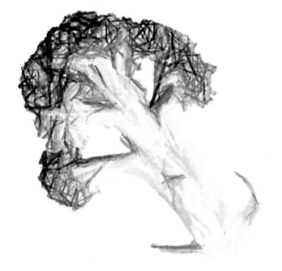

Bite-Size Vegetable Patties

INGREDIENTS

1 cup	TVP (Textured Vegetable Protein)
1 small	onion
1 clove	garlic
1 Tbsp	fresh thyme
1 pinch	dried sage
1 tsp	dried basil
1 bundle	scallions, diced
2 Tbsp	nutritional yeast
½ cup	whole wheat bread crumbs
2 Tbsp	vegetable oil
2 cup	filtered water
½ tsp	cayenne pepper
	pie shells (See recipe)

DIRECTIONS

1. Sauté in vegetable oil, onion, garlic, thyme, sage, basil and scallions.

2. Add TVP and mix for 1 minute.

3. Pour 2 cups water on mixture and let cook for 10 minutes.

4. Add carrots, bread crumbs, cayenne pepper, nutritional yeast, and salt or Spike.

5. Turn off stove and allow mixture to cool. Mixture should be soft and not too dry. If dry, add a little more water.

6. Cut pastry with glass. Spoon mixture onto half of pastry and fold over.

7. Press down sides with fork. Add holes to top of pastry. Press fork teeth into top of pastry once and bake.

8. Place on a greased cookie sheet and bake for 10 to 15 minutes at 350F.

Vegetable Fritters

INGREDIENTS

1 cup	chickpea flour
1 tsp	salt
1 pinch	cayenne pepper
1 small	onion
1 small	yellow squash
1 small	zucchini
1 head	cauliflower
1 head	broccoli
1 tsp	ginger powder
½ to 2/3 cup	water
2 cups	peanut oil
2 med	carrots cut in 2-inch strips
1 heaping tsp	cumin powder

DIRECTIONS

1. Cut broccoli and cauliflower into florets and remaining vegetables into 2-inch strips.

2. Make a thick batter using all ingredients except vegetable pieces.

3. Beat briskly to remove any lumps. Consistency should be like cake batter.

4. Heat oil and dip vegetable pieces.

5. Fry a few at a time in hot oil and serve.

Ja Coco Fritters

Coco is a tuberous food. It is also called edows in Guyana and coco in Jamaica.

INGREDIENTS

2 to 3 small	cocos
1 Tbsp	flour
½ tsp	bicarbonate of soda or ½ tsp baking powder
2 stalks	scallions
½ tsp	salt
1 pinch	pepper

DIRECTIONS

1. Wash and peel cocos.
2. Wash again, grate finely and mix all ingredients. Beat well.
3. Drop by spoonful into very hot oil. Fry until golden brown.
4. Drain and serve at once.

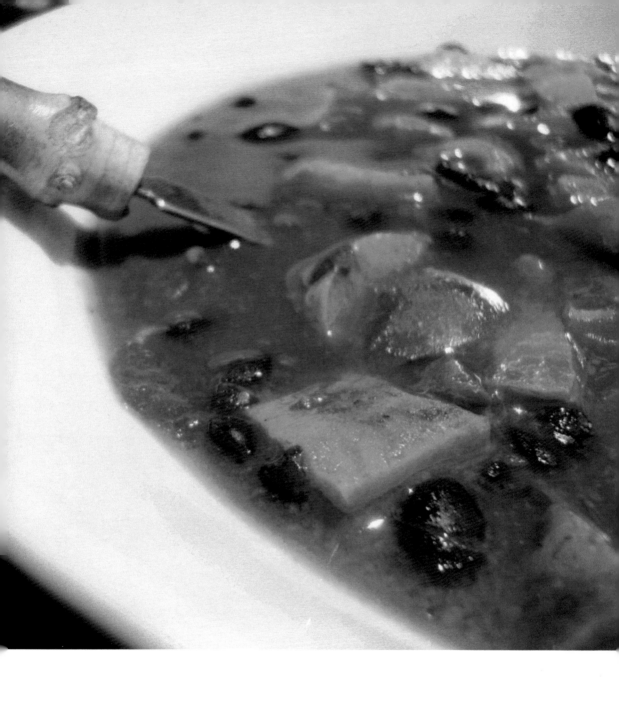

BLACK BEAN SOUP (p. 68)

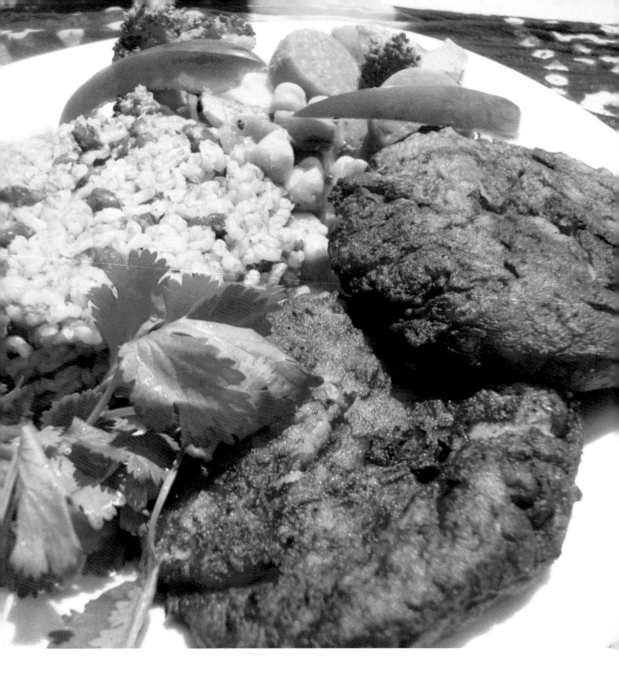

BROWN RICE AND PEAS (p. 59)
CHICKPEA PATTIES (p. 52)
CURRIED VEGETABLES (p.57)

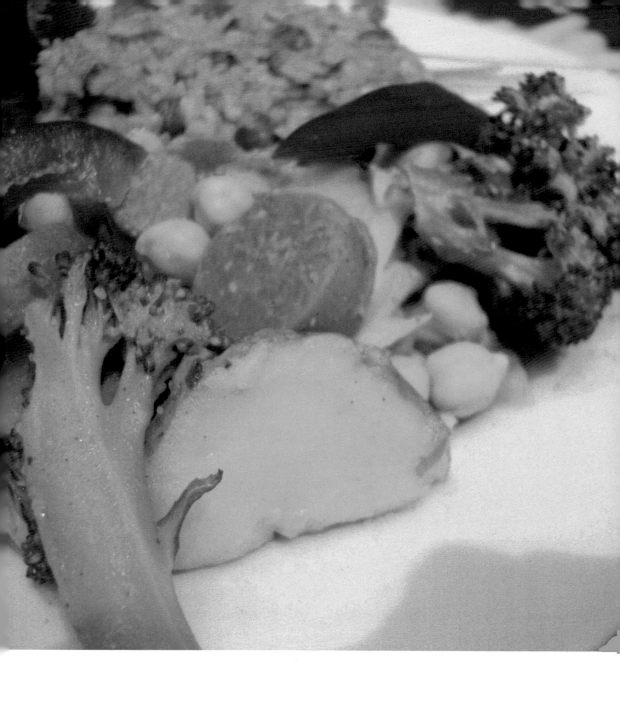

CURRIED VEGETABLES (p. 57)

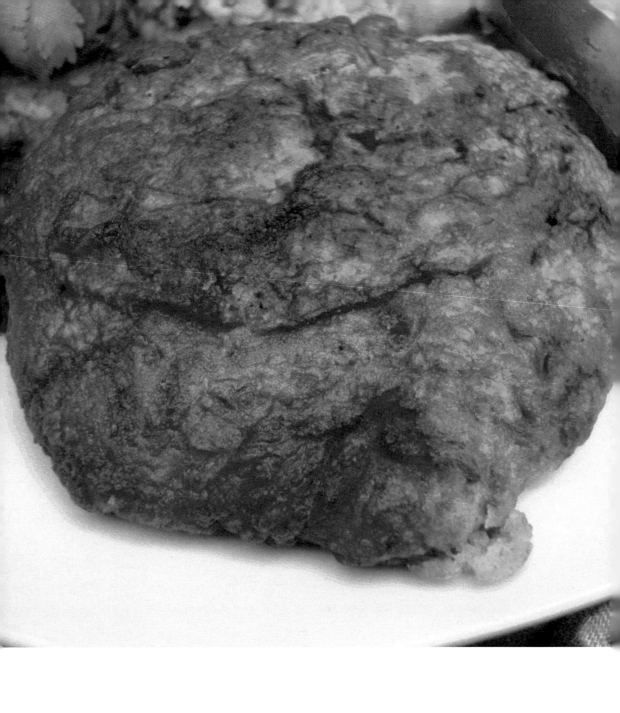

CHICKPEA PATTIES (p. 52)

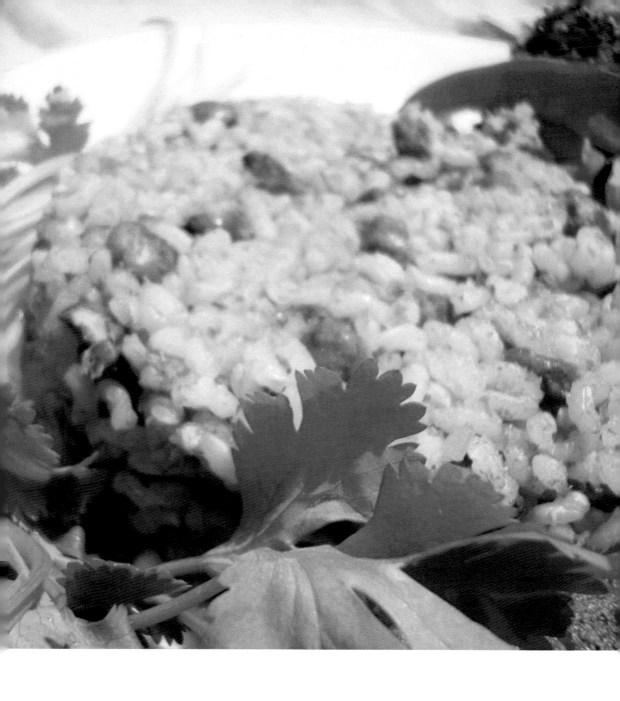

BROWN RICE AND PEAS (p. 59)

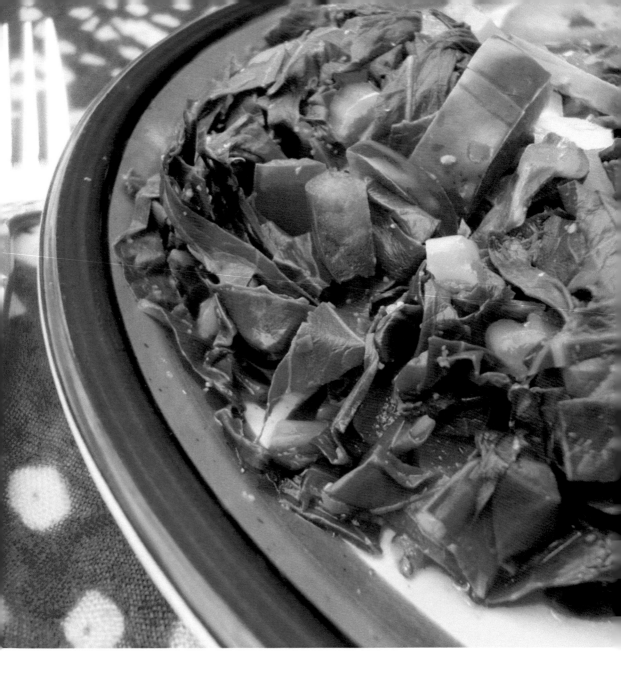

SPICY GREENS (p. 33)

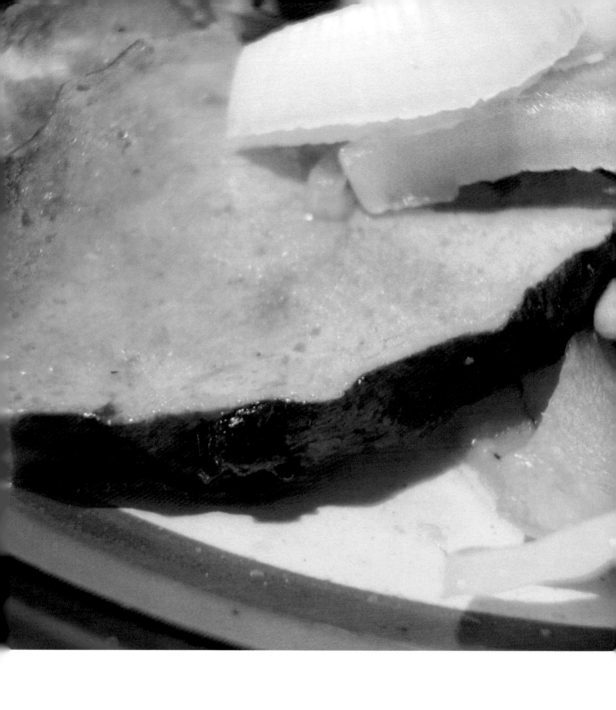

UNFISH
(available in restaurant)

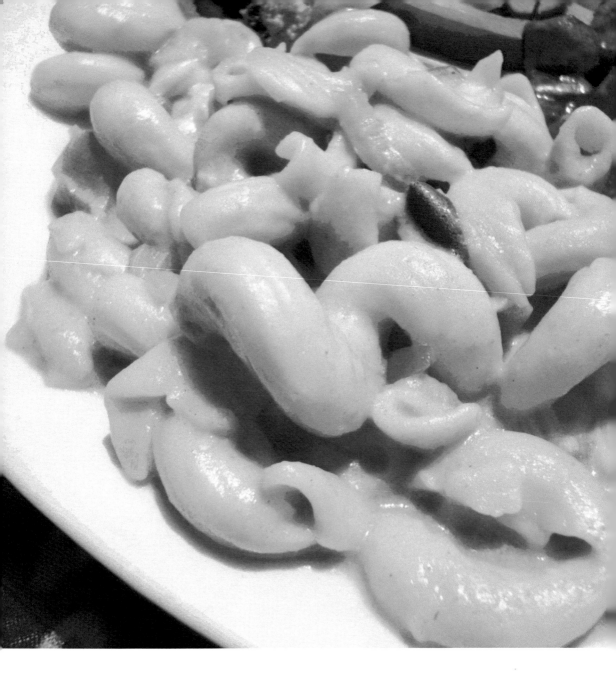

VEGAN MACARONI UNCHEESE (p. 51)

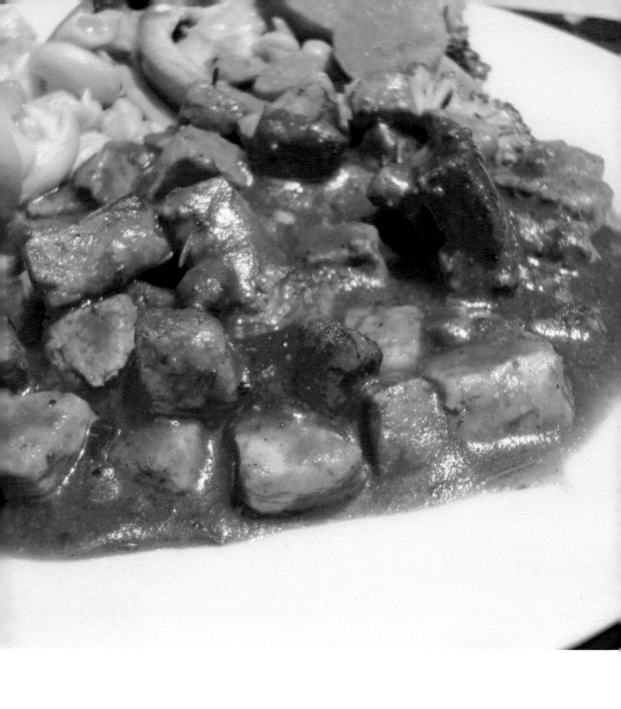

BBQ TOFU (p. 49)

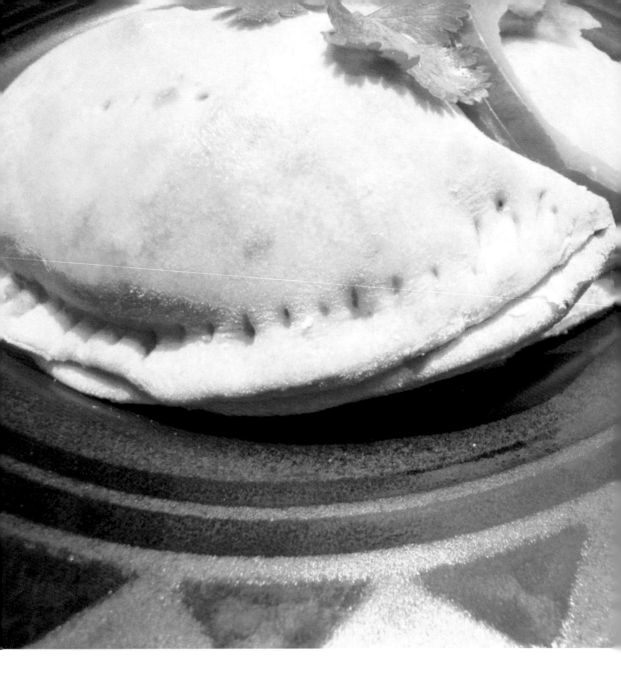

VEGETABLE PATTIES
(available in restaurant)

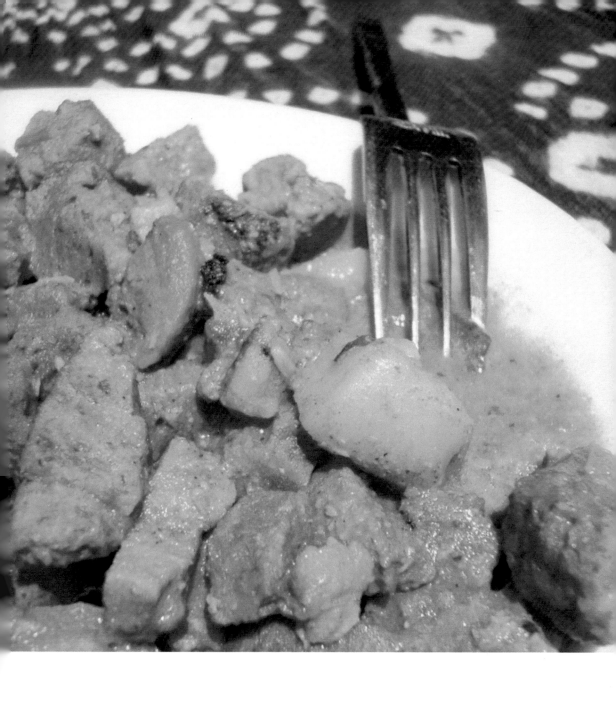

CURRIED UNGOAT
(available in restaurant)

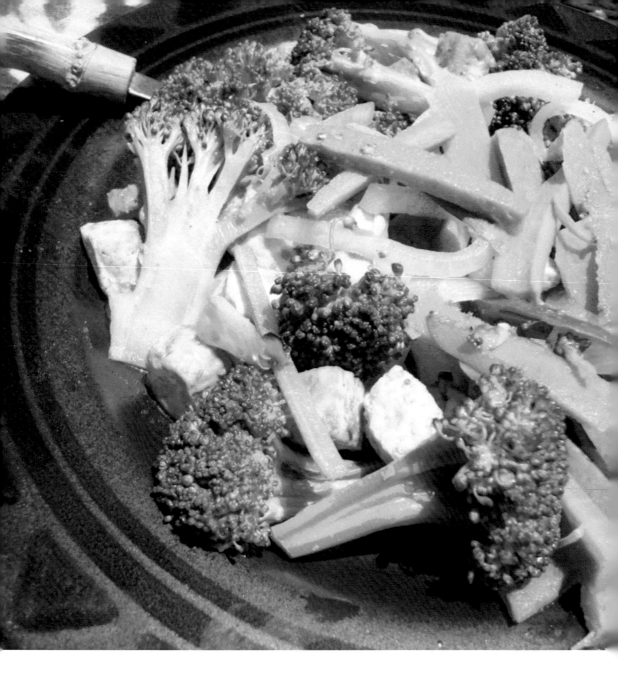

SAUTEED TOFU AND VEGETABLES
(available in restaurant)

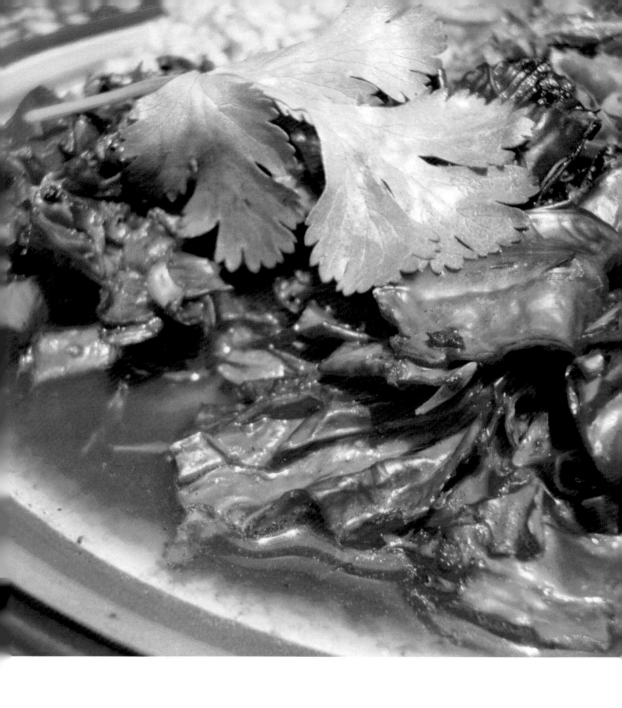

JERK BEAN CURD
(available in restaurant)

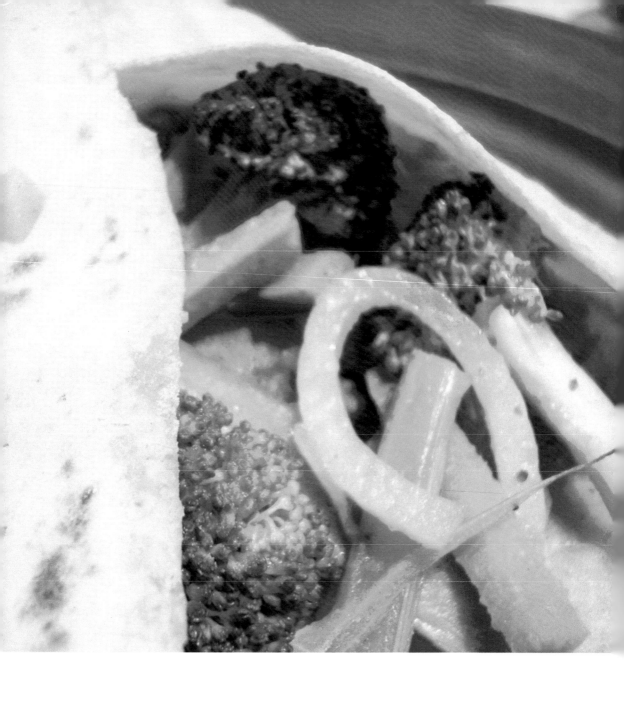

ROTI WRAP WITH CURRIED UNGOAT, SAUTEED VEGETABLES AND RICE
(WRAPS CAN BE STUFFED WITH FOOD OF CHOICE)
(available in restaurant)

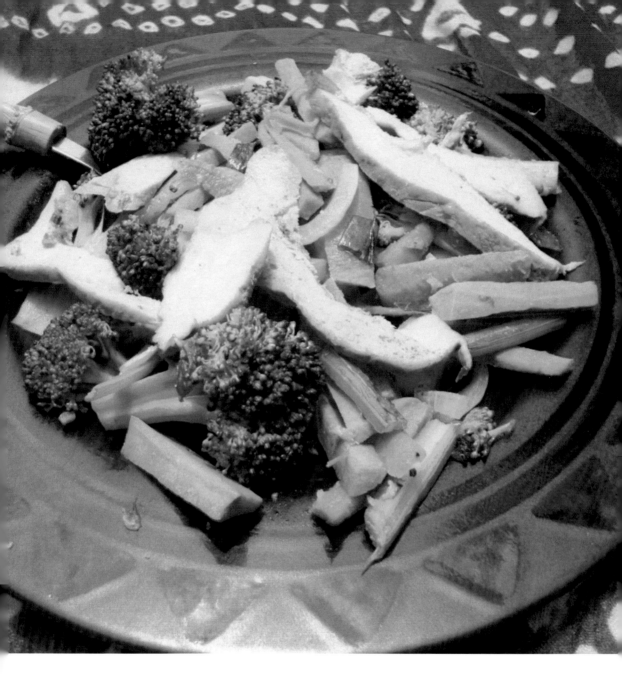

UNCHICKEN WITH VEGETABLES
(available in restaurant)

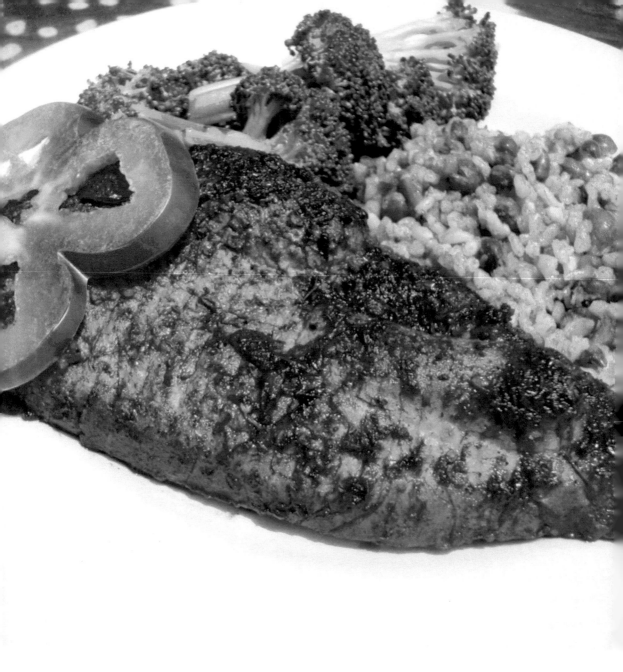

JERK UNCHICKEN (available in restaurant)
BROWN RICE AND PEAS (p. 59)
BROCCOLI (available in restaurant)

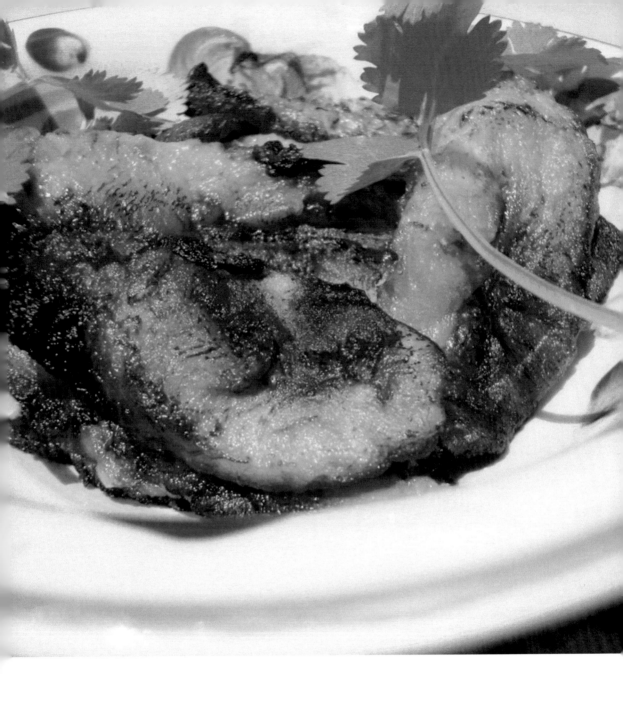

FRIED PLANTAINS
(available in restaurant)

ABOUT THE AUTHOR

Princess Rowena Daly-Dixon is the owner/operator of Healthful Essence Vegetarian Restaurant, located at 875 York Avenue S.W., Atlanta, GA 30310. She has been a staple in the health-conscious and in the surrounding Atlanta community for over 15 years. She

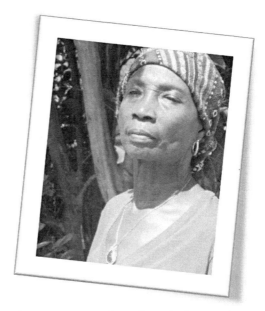

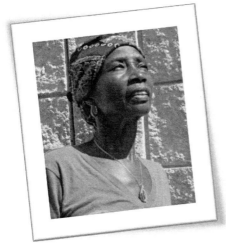

has been preparing food since the age of nine and has since studied under such greats as Dr. Ignatius Foster, founder of Microcosmic Science. These studies encouraged the formation and maintenance of

a healthy lifestyle through the preparation of healthy foods. She is deeply committed to healthy living by using her culinary skills to prepare healthy and nutritious cuisine.

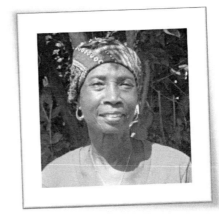

INDEX

THIS BOOK MAKES A GREAT GIFT!

Healthful Essence Cookbook:
Caribbean-Style Vegan Vegetarian Meals
One book $18.95 each plus $2.50 shipping & handling
(Georgia residents add 7% sales tax)
TOTAL $ _____

2 or more books $15.00 each plus $2.50 shipping & handling for each book
(Georgia residents add 7% sales tax)
TOTAL $ _____

Make checks or money orders payable to:
Princess Rowena Daly-Dixon

Return this form with payment enclosed to:
Princess Rowena Daly-Dixon
875 York Avenue, SW
Atlanta, GA 30310

Please send my order to:

Name: _____

Address: _____

City, State, Zip: _____

Phone: _____

Email: _____

Thank you for your order!

You can also order online at www.healthfullessence.com,
or in our restaurant located at 875 York Avenue, SW, Atlanta, GA 30310!

HEALTHFUL ESSENCE COOKBOOK
Caribbean-Style Vegan Vegetarian Meals
ISBN-10: 061551314X
ISBN-13: 978-0-615-51314-0

$18.95
ISBN 978-0-615-51314-0

51895>

9 780615 513140